Instant Pot Duo Crisp Cookbook

Quick and Easy Instant Pot Air Fryer Crisp Recipes from Breakfast to Dessert

Louise Davidson

All rights reserved © 2021 by Louise Davidson and The Cookbook Publisher. No part of this All rights reserved © 2020 by Louise Davidson and The Cookbook Publisher. No part of this publication or the information in it may be quoted from or reproduced in any form by means such as printing, scanning, photocopying, or otherwise without prior written permission of the copyright holder.

This book is presented solely for motivational and informational purposes. The author and the publisher do not hold any responsibility for errors, omissions, or contrary interpretation of the subject matter herein.

The recipes provided in this book are for informational purposes only and are not intended to provide dietary advice. A medical practitioner should be consulted before making any changes in diet. Additionally, recipes' cooking times may require adjustment depending on the age and quality of appliances. Readers are strongly urged to take all precautions to ensure ingredients are fully cooked to avoid the dangers of foodborne illnesses. The recipes and suggestions provided in this book are solely the opinions of the author. The author and publisher do not take any responsibility for any consequences that may result due to following the instructions provided in this book.

All the nutritional information contained in this book is provided for informational purposes only. This information is based on the specific brands, ingredients, and measurements used to make the recipe, and therefore the nutritional information is an estimate, and in no way is intended to be a guarantee of the actual nutritional value of the recipe made in the reader's home. The author and the publisher will not be responsible for any damages resulting in your reliance on the nutritional information. The best method to obtain an accurate count of the nutritional value in the recipe is to calculate the information with your specific brands, ingredients, and measurements.

ISBN: 9798706469757

Printed in the United States

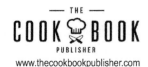

www.thecookbookpublisher.com

CONTENTS

INTRODUCTION 1

APPETIZERS AND SNACKS 5

CHICKEN AND POULTRY 15

BEEF, PORK, AND LAMB 37

FISH AND SEAFOOD 57

MEATLESS 67

SIDES 79

DESSERTS 89

RECIPE INDEX 93

APPENDIX 95

INTRODUCTION

The perfect air fried crust of those juicy ribs beats everything. That delicious fall-off-the-bone feel is simply irresistible. The next generation Instant Pot Duo Crisp is designed for the ultimate convenience to cook fresh and healthy meals at home.

Instead of just one pressure lid, this new model offers cooking convenience with two lids (a pressure lid and an air fryer lid). Now, with just one Instant Pot, you can cook both pressure cooked and air fried recipes. Not only that, but this new model also allows you to cook all your favorite baked, roasted, and broiled cuisines with additional cooking functions.

Foods that are air fried with the Instant Pot Duo Crisp are healthy and low in carbohydrates as it uses revolutionary air frying technology that requires less oil to cook foods. Roasted and baked recipes are also healthier with the use of fresh and nutritious foods.

In the mood for a juicy steak, BBQ drumsticks, fall-off-the-bone lamb chops, or tender crisp chicken wings? Wait no longer; bring home an Instant Pot Duo Crisp and postpone all your other plans to gear up for an amazing culinary feast.

Beginner's Guide to Using the Instant Pot Duo Crisp

With the assistance of 11-in–1 modern cooking functions, the Instant Pot Duo Crisp takes away your cooking concerns. Anything you want to cook, you just have to press a few buttons and you are all set to enjoy delicious meals with your whole family. Operating the Instant Pot Duo Crisp is very easy and comfortable. As compared to previous pressure cooking models, this new model is designed to add versatility to your meal plan with two removable lids (pressure lid and air fryer lid) and added cooking functions (Air Fry, Bake, Roast, Broil, Dehydrate).

While you can cook all standard pressure cooked meals using the pressure lid, the air fryer lid is for preparing recipes that use the Air Fry, Bake, Roast, Broil, and Dehydrate functions. The essential parts of the newly designed Instant Pot Duo Crisp are:

- Main unit
- Main inner cooking pot
- Multi-level air frying basket
- Pressure lid
- Air fryer lid
- Steam rack
- Broil/dehydrate tray
- Protective pad and storage cover

Cooking with the Air Fryer Lid

The Instant Pot Duo Crisp comes with a separate multi-level air frying basket to hold foods. The air fryer lid is used to air fry, bake, broil, roast, or dehydrate. It is recommended to grease the basket to avoid food burning and sticking to the bottom surface.

First, you add the prepared ingredients to the basket. Then you place this basket inside the main cooking pot. After that, you place the air fryer lid on top of the Instant Pot Duo Crisp and lock it. Now you are all set to start cooking. Select your desired cooking function, set the temperature level and timer, and press START to initiate cooking.

When using the Air Fry mode, the Instant Pot Duo Crisp will indicate TURN FOOD halfway through the set cooking time. At this point, you can either turn the food or just shake the basket. It helps to cook the ingredients evenly. However, not all recipes need the food to be turned. If you do nothing, the unit will resume cooking for the remaining time. After the cooking time is over, press CANCEL, open the air fryer lid and enjoy your freshly prepared meal.

Cooking with the Pressure Lid

The pressure lid functions in the same way as any other Instant Pot model. With pressure cooking, you add the ingredients directly into the main inner pot instead of the air frying basket. Just add the ingredients, lock the pressure lid on top, select the cooking mode (LOW, MEDIUM, or HIGH), set the timer, and press START to initiate cooking.

Multiple Lid Cooking

Many recipes use pressure cooking followed by air frying, roasting, broiling, or baking. For such recipes, you have to use both the pressure lid and the air fryer lid. In most cases, a recipe calls for transferring pressure cooked food into the air frying basket and continuing with the second part of cooking using the air fryer lid. The process remains the same as mentioned above for the respective cooking functions.

Experience a whole new world of Instant Pot cooking with the technologically advanced Instant Pot Duo Crisp. The book covers an exclusive collection of 50 tender crisp recipes using the air fryer lid. This complete air fryer cookbook provides healthy, fresh, and fast cuisine for everyone with exclusive chapters covering appetizers, snacks, and sides; chicken and poultry; beef, pork, and lamb; fish and seafood; meatless meals; and desserts.

It's time to open the pot of infinite possibilities and explore the secret of guilt-free Instant Pot Duo Crisp cooking. Let's get started!

APPETIZERS AND SNACKS

Crispy Sausage Bites

Serves 18 meatballs | Prep. time 5–10 minutes | Cooking time 20 minutes

Ingredients
½ pound uncooked maple pork sausage, casings removed
2 ounces cream cheese
1 cup baking mix
1 cup shredded cheddar cheese

Directions
1. In a mixing bowl, combine the cream cheese and sausage.
2. Mix in the baking mix.
3. Prepare 18 meatballs from the mixture.
4. Add 1 cup of water to the inner cooking pot.
5. Place the air frying basket inside the pot. Grease the basket with some vegetable oil or cooking spray.
6. Add half of the meatballs to the basket. Arrange the broiling tray in the basket and place the remaining meatballs on top.
7. Place the pressure lid on top in a lock position.
8. Press PRESSURE. Select HIGH-PRESSURE mode and set the timer to 5 minutes.
9. Press START. After cooking time is over quick release the pressure.
10. Press CANCEL and take out the air frying basket; drain the liquid.
11. Return the basket to the inner cooking pot.
12. Place the air fryer lid on top; press AIR FRY. Set temperature to 360°F and timer to 8 minutes.

13. Press START. When the Instant Pot Duo Crisp indicates TURN FOOD, do nothing.
14. Serve warm.

Nutrition (per meatball)
Calories 68, fat 4 g, total carbs 5 g,
Protein 3 g, sodium 117 mg

French Fries

Serves 4 | Prep. time 5–10 minutes | Cooking time 20 minutes

Ingredients
2 large potatoes, sliced into ¼-inch sticks
3 tablespoons canola or olive oil
1 teaspoon paprika
1 teaspoon pepper
1 teaspoon salt

Directions
1. In a mixing bowl, combine the potatoes and olive oil. Mix until the potatoes are coated well.
2. Season with paprika, salt, and pepper.
3. Arrange the steam rack inside the dry inner pot of the Instant Pot Duo Crisp.
4. Place the air frying basket on the steam rack.
5. Place the coated potatoes inside the basket.
6. Place the air fryer lid on top; press AIR FRY. Set temperature to 375°F and timer to 20 minutes.
7. Press START. When the Instant Pot Duo Crisp indicates TURN FOOD, flip the fries and continue to cook for the remaining time.
8. Serve warm.

Nutrition (per serving)
Calories 266, fat 11 g, total carbs 34 g,
Protein 5 g, sodium 602 mg

Cauliflower Crisp Bites

Serves 6–8 | Prep. time 5–10 minutes | Cooking time 8 minutes

Ingredients
1 head of cauliflower, cut into florets
1 egg
⅓ cup shredded mozzarella cheese
⅓ cup shredded sharp cheddar cheese
½ cup chopped parsley
1 cup Italian breadcrumbs
3 chopped scallions
2 cloves garlic, minced

Directions
1. In a blender, blend the cauliflower florets to a rice-like consistency.
2. In a mixing bowl, beat the egg. Add the cauliflower mix, cheeses, breadcrumbs, pepper, salt, garlic, and scallions.
3. Make 15 small patties from the mixture. Coat them with cooking spray.
4. Arrange the air frying basket inside the dry inner pot of the Instant Pot Duo Crisp. Grease the basket with some vegetable oil or cooking spray.
5. Place the patties inside the basket.
6. Place the air fryer lid on top; press AIR FRY. Set temperature to 390°F and timer to 8 minutes.
7. Press START. When the Instant Pot Duo Crisp indicates TURN FOOD, flip the patties and continue to cook for the remaining time.
8. Serve warm.

Nutrition (per serving)
Calories 239, fat 18 g, total carbs 30 g,
Protein 6 g, sodium 523 mg

Prosciutto Wrapped Dates

Serves 12 | Prep. time 5 minutes | Cooking time 3 minutes

Ingredients
10 ounces Medjool dates, pitted and halved
6 ounces brie cheese
3 ounces sliced prosciutto, cut into strips
Honey (optional)

Directions
1. Remove the rind from the cheese.
2. Stuff the date halves with cheese.
3. Wrap each date half with a prosciutto slice.
4. Arrange the air frying basket inside the dry inner pot of the Instant Pot Duo Crisp. Grease the basket with some vegetable oil or cooking spray.
5. Place the wrapped dates inside the basket.
6. Place the air fryer lid on top; press AIR FRY. Set temperature to 400°F and timer to 3 minutes.
7. Press START. When the Instant Pot Duo Crisp indicates TURN FOOD, do nothing.
8. Serve warm with some honey on top (optional).

Nutrition (per serving)
Calories 123, fat 5 g, total carbs 16 g,
Protein 5 g, sodium 231 mg

Fried Cheesy Pickles

Serves 4 | Prep. time 5–10 minutes | Cooking time 8 minutes

Ingredients
2 eggs
½ cup Italian-style bread crumbs
½ cup panko bread crumbs
¼ cup Parmesan cheese
1 tablespoon garlic powder
1 teaspoon Cajun seasoning
1–2 cups dill pickles, sliced and drained

Directions
1. In a mixing bowl, beat the eggs.
2. In another mixing bowl, combine the crumbs, cheese, cheese, garlic powder, and Cajun seasoning.
3. Dip the dill slices first in the eggs and then in the crumb mixture to coat evenly.
4. Arrange the air frying basket inside the dry inner pot of the Instant Pot Duo Crisp. Grease the basket with some vegetable oil or cooking spray.
5. Place the pickle slices inside the basket and spray them with cooking spray.
6. Place the air fryer lid on top; press AIR FRY. Set temperature to 360°F and timer to 10 minutes.
7. Press START. When the Instant Pot Duo Crisp indicates TURN FOOD, flip the pickle slices and continue to cook for the remaining time.
8. Serve warm.

Nutrition (per serving)
Calories 150, fat 5 g, total carbs 17g,
Protein 8 g, sodium 700 mg

Falafel

Serves 6 | Prep. time 5–10 minutes | Cooking time 10 minutes

Ingredients
2 tablespoons tahini paste
2 teaspoons cumin powder
2 tablespoons minced cilantro leaves
1 tablespoon minced parsley
1 tablespoon dill
2 tablespoons lime or lemon juice
1 cup cooked chickpeas
2 cloves garlic, minced
½ onion, finely chopped
¼ cup flour
2 tablespoons sesame oil
Salt to taste

Directions
1. In a blender, blend the tahini, cumin, cilantro, parsley, dill, lime juice, chickpeas, garlic, onion, and salt into a smooth paste.
2. Mix in the flour. Prepare small patties from the mixture.
3. Arrange the air frying basket inside the dry inner pot of the Instant Pot Duo Crisp. Grease the basket with some sesame oil.
4. Place the patties inside the basket.
5. Place the air fryer lid on top; press AIR FRY. Set temperature to 350°F and timer to 10 minutes.
6. Press START. When the Instant Pot Duo Crisp indicates TURN FOOD, turn the patties and continue to cook for the remaining time.
7. Serve warm.

Nutrition (per serving)
Calories 206, fat 7 g, total carbs 31 g,
Protein 8 g, sodium 1216 mg

Chicken Kebabs

Serves 4 | Prep. time 15–20 minutes | Cooking time 15 minutes

Ingredients
1 pound boneless skinless chicken thighs cut into 2-inch cubes
1 tablespoon vegetable oil
½ cup red onion, cut into 2-inch pieces
½ cup green bell pepper, cut into 2-inch pieces
½ cup red bell pepper, cut into 2-inch pieces
Lime wedges and onion rounds to garnish

Marinade
½ cup Greek yogurt
¾ tablespoon grated ginger
¾ tablespoon minced garlic
1 tablespoon lime juice
½ teaspoon ground turmeric
1 teaspoon garam masala or spice mix
1 teaspoon coriander powder
½ tablespoon dried fenugreek leaves
Salt and red chili powder to taste

Directions
1. In a mixing bowl, combine the marinade ingredients.
2. Add the chicken and coat well.
3. Cover with foil and refrigerate for 30 minutes–8 hours.
4. Add the bell peppers, onions, and oil; mix well.
5. Thread the chicken, peppers, and onions alternately onto skewers. Lightly brush the skewers with some oil.
6. Arrange the air frying basket inside the dry inner pot of the Instant Pot Duo Crisp. Grease the basket with some vegetable oil or cooking spray.

7. Place the skewers inside the basket. Cook in batches.
8. Place the air fryer lid on top; press AIR FRY. Set temperature to 400°F and timer to 16 minutes.
9. Press START. When the Instant Pot Duo Crisp indicates TURN FOOD, flip the skewers and continue to cook for the remaining time until the chicken is evenly charred.
10. Add the onion rings and lemon wedges to decorate; serve with your choice of dip.

Nutrition (per serving)
Calories 337, fat 24 g, total carbs 9 g,
Protein 21 g, sodium 622 mg

CHICKEN AND POULTRY

Chicken Broccoli Casserole

Serves 8 | Prep. time 5–10 minutes | Cooking time 25 minutes

Ingredients
3 cups shredded chicken
¾ pound egg noodles
½ large onions
½ cup chopped carrots
¼ cup frozen peas
¼ cup frozen broccoli pieces
2 stalks celery, chopped
5 cups chicken broth
1 teaspoon garlic powder
Salt and pepper to taste
1 cup shredded cheddar cheese
1 package French's Original Crispy Fried Onions
¼ cup sour cream
1 can cream of chicken and mushroom soup

Directions
1. Add chicken and veggies to the dry inner pot of the Instant Pot Duo Crisp.
2. Add the garlic powder, salt and pepper, and broth; stir with a wooden spatula.
3. Mix in the egg noodles.
4. Place the pressure lid on top in a lock position.
5. Press PRESSURE. Select HIGH-PRESSURE mode and set the timer to 4 minutes.
6. Press START. After cooking time is over quick release the pressure.

7. Mix in the cheese, sour cream, soup, and ⅓ of the French's onions.
8. Scatter the remaining French's onions on top.
9. Place the air fryer lid on top; press AIR FRY. Set temperature to 400°F and timer to 5 minutes.
10. When the Instant Pot Duo Crisp indicates TURN FOOD, do nothing. Cook until onions are golden brown.
11. Serve warm.

Nutrition (per serving)
Calories 300, fat 17 g, total carbs 17 g,
Protein 20 g, sodium 877 mg

Chicken Poutine

Serves 4 | Prep. time 5–10 minutes | Cooking time 50 minutes

Ingredients
2 pounds potatoes, cut into 1-inch wedges
¼ teaspoon pepper
¼ teaspoon salt
2 tablespoons canola oil
1 cup of shredded cooked chicken
1 cup cheese curds
½ cup shredded aged cheddar cheese
¼ cup crumbled blue cheese
⅓ cup buffalo wing sauce
½ cup ranch dressing
2 cups carrot and celery sticks

Directions
1. Season the potato wedges with salt and pepper.
2. Arrange the air frying basket inside the dry inner pot of the Instant Pot Duo Crisp. Grease the basket with some vegetable oil or cooking spray.
3. Place the wedges inside the basket and drizzle with olive oil. Cook in two batches.
4. Place the air fryer lid on top; press AIR FRY. Set temperature to 400°F and timer to 22–24 minutes.
5. Press START. When the Instant Pot Duo Crisp indicates TURN FOOD, shake the basket and continue to cook for the remaining time until wedges are golden brown.
6. Transfer the wedges to a serving plate; add the chicken and top with the cheese curd, cheddar, and blue cheese.
7. Top with the buffalo wing sauce and 2 tablespoons of the ranch dressing.

8. Serve with carrot and celery sticks and the remaining ranch dressing as a dip.

Nutrition (per serving)
Calories 640, fat 39 g, total carbs 47 g,
Protein 27 g, sodium 1450 mg

Orange Roast Chicken

Serves 4 | Prep. time 5–10 minutes | Cooking time 45 minutes

Ingredients
2 teaspoons dried oregano
2 teaspoons chili powder
2 teaspoons ground cumin
2 teaspoons coarse salt
1 teaspoon brown sugar
1 teaspoon pepper
1 (3-pound) whole chicken
2 bay leaves
1 small onion, quartered
¼ cup lime juice
¼ cup lemon juice
¼ cup orange juice
¼ cup olive oil (divided)
½ Serrano chili pepper, seeded and diced
1 tablespoon Dijon mustard
4 cloves garlic, minced
2 cups low-sodium chicken broth

Directions
1. In a mixing bowl, combine the oregano, chili powder, cumin, salt, brown sugar, and pepper.
2. Rub the spice mix over the chicken and inside its cavity.
3. Add the chicken, onion and bay leave to a Ziploc bag.
4. In another mixing bowl, combine the lime juice, lemon juice, orange juice, chili pepper, mustard, garlic, and 3 tablespoons of the olive oil.
5. Pour the mixture inside the bag and shake to coat the chicken.
6. Refrigerate for 4 hours–overnight.

7. Remove chicken from bag; reserve marinade.
8. To the dry inner cooking pot of the Instant Pot Duo Crisp, add the reserved marinade, broth, and chicken (breast side down); stir with a wooden spatula.
9. Place the pressure lid on top in a lock position.
10. Press PRESSURE. Select HIGH-PRESSURE mode and set the timer to 20 minutes.
11. Press START. After cooking time is over quick release the pressure.
12. Remove the chicken and pat dry. Empty the pot.
13. Coat the chicken with the remaining olive oil.
14. Arrange the air frying basket inside the dry inner pot of the Instant Pot Duo Crisp. Place the chicken inside the basket (breast side up).
15. Place the air fryer lid on top; press ROAST. Set temperature to 400°F and timer to 25 minutes.
16. Press START. Cook until the food thermometer indicates 165°F.
17. Slice and serve warm.

Nutrition (per serving)
Calories 560, fat 38 g, total carbs 11 g,
Protein 45 g, sodium 1540 mg

BBQ Drumsticks

Serves 4 | Prep. time 5–10 minutes | Cooking time 25 minutes

Ingredients
6–8 chicken drumsticks

BBQ Mix
1 tablespoon salt
¼ cup sweet paprika
1 teaspoon celery salt
1 teaspoon garlic powder
1 teaspoon ground cumin
1 teaspoon dry mustard
1 teaspoon cayenne pepper
3½ teaspoons pepper

Directions
1. Pour ¾ cup of water into the dry inner cooking pot of the Instant Pot Duo Crisp; arrange the steam rack.
2. Place the chicken drumsticks over the steam rack.
3. Place the pressure lid on top in a lock position.
4. Press PRESSURE. Select HIGH-PRESSURE mode and set the timer to 20 minutes.
5. Press START. After cooking time is over natural release the pressure.
6. Remove the drumsticks. In a mixing bowl, combine the BBQ mix ingredients.
7. Rub the drumsticks with BBQ mix and arrange them on parchment paper.
8. Place the drumsticks inside the pot.
9. Place the air fryer lid on top; press BROIL. Select HIGH-PRESSURE mode and set the timer to 2 minutes.
10. Cook until drumsticks are evenly brown. After cooking time is over quick release the pressure.

11. Serve warm.

Nutrition (per serving)
Calories 179, fat 4 g, total carbs 12 g,
Protein 19 g, sodium 1658 mg

Seasoned Whole Chicken

Serves 4 | Prep. time 5–10 minutes | Cooking time 45 minutes

Ingredients
1 teaspoon garlic powder
1 teaspoon onion powder
1 teaspoon paprika
1 teaspoon Italian seasoning
2 tablespoons Montreal steak seasoning (or salt and pepper to taste)
1 whole chicken
2 tablespoons olive oil spray
1½ cups chicken broth

Directions
1. In a mixing bowl, combine the seasonings.
2. Coat the chicken with a small amount of seasoning.
3. Add the chicken and broth to the dry inner pot of the Instant Pot Duo Crisp. Place the pressure lid on top in a lock position.
4. Press PRESSURE. Select HIGH-PRESSURE mode and set the timer to 25 minutes.
5. Press START. After cooking time is over quick release the pressure.
6. Remove the liquid. Empty and dry the inner pot.
7. Arrange the air frying basket inside the dry inner pot of the Instant Pot Duo Crisp. Place the chicken inside the basket. Coat with half of the seasoning and half of the olive oil.
8. Place the air fryer lid on top; press AIR FRY. Set temperature to 400°F and timer to 20 minutes. 204C
9. Press START. When the Instant Pot Duo Crisp indicates TURN FOOD, flip the chicken and coat with the remaining seasoning and olive oil. Continue to

cook for the remaining time until the food thermometer indicates 160°F. 1c
10. Carve chicken and serve warm.

Nutrition (per serving)
Calories 441, fat 28 g, total carbs 4 g,
Protein 42 g, sodium 1192 mg

Red Hot Chicken Wings

Serves 12 | Prep. time 5–10 minutes | Cooking time 40 minutes

Ingredients
12–24 party-style chicken wings
1 tablespoon olive oil
1 cup chicken broth or water
¼ cup butter
½ cup red hot sauce
¼ teaspoon Worcestershire sauce
1 tablespoon white vinegar
¼ teaspoon cayenne pepper
⅛ teaspoon garlic powder
Seasoned salt to taste
Ranch dressing or blue cheese for dipping
Celery

Directions
1. Add the broth/water and chicken wings to the dry inner cooking pot of the Instant Pot Duo Crisp; stir with a wooden spatula.
2. Place the pressure lid on top in a lock position.
3. Press PRESSURE. Select HIGH-PRESSURE mode and set the timer to 10 minutes.
4. Press START. After cooking time is over quick release the pressure. Empty the inner pot.
5. Coat the chicken wings with olive oil. Season with salt and pepper. Set aside.
6. Add the butter, Worcestershire sauce, hot sauce, cayenne pepper, vinegar, and garlic powder to the inner pot.
7. Press SAUTE; stir-cook until the mixture starts to bubble. Set the sauce aside.

8. Arrange the air frying basket inside the dry inner pot of the Instant Pot Duo Crisp. Grease the basket with some vegetable oil or cooking spray.
9. Place the chicken wings inside the basket.
10. Place the air fryer lid on top; press AIR FRY. Set temperature to 400°F and timer to 20 minutes.
11. Press START. When the Instant Pot Duo Crisp indicates TURN FOOD, flip the chicken wings, spray them with more cooking spray if needed, and continue to cook for the remaining time.
12. Serve warm with warm sauce on top, celery, and dip of your choice.

Nutrition (per serving)
Calories 463, fat 40 g, total carbs 10 g,
Protein 16 g, sodium 1647 mg

Turkey Meatloaf

Serves 6 | Prep. time 5–10 minutes | Cooking time 45 minutes

Ingredients
2 tablespoons butter
1 small onion, minced
3 garlic cloves, minced
1 pound ground turkey
1 cup Ritz crackers or plain breadcrumbs, finely crushed
2 teaspoons Worcestershire sauce
1 egg
Salt and pepper to taste
1 teaspoon garlic powder
¾ pound green beans, trimmed
1 tablespoon olive oil
3 tablespoons BBQ sauce

Directions
1. Add the butter and onions to the dry inner pot of the Instant Pot Duo Crisp.
2. Press SAUTE; stir-cook for 3–4 minutes until softened and translucent.
3. Add the garlic and stir cook for 1 minute more. Clean the inner pot.
4. Set aside the onion mixture in a large bowl.
5. Add the crumbs, turkey, Worcestershire sauce, egg, salt, and pepper.
6. Line an 8×4-inch loaf pan with foil.
7. Add the turkey mixture and press gently.
8. Pull out the foil along with the turkey mixture. Place it over a steak rack.
9. Place the rack inside the inner pot. Pour in 1 cup of water.
10. Place the pressure lid on top in a lock position.

11. Press PRESSURE. Select HIGH-PRESSURE mode and set the timer to 20 minutes.
12. Press START. After cooking time is over natural release the pressure.
13. Remove the meatloaf and empty the inner pot.
14. In a mixing bowl, combine the garlic powder, ¾ teaspoon salt, ¼ teaspoon pepper, green beans, and olive oil.
15. Brush the meatloaf with BBQ sauce.
16. Arrange the air frying basket inside the dry inner pot of the Instant Pot Duo Crisp. Place the meatloaf inside the basket.
17. Arrange the broiling tray and arrange the green beans over it.
18. Place the air fryer lid on top; press AIR FRY. Set temperature to 370°F and timer to 8 minutes.
19. Press START. When the Instant Pot Duo Crisp indicates TURN FOOD, toss the green beans and continue to cook for the remaining time until a food thermometer in the meatloaf indicates 160°F.
20. Slice and serve warm with green beans.

Nutrition (per serving)
Calories 290, fat 17 g, total carbs 20 g,
Protein 18 g, sodium 468 mg

Parmesan Chicken Roast

Serves 6 | Prep. time 5–10 minutes | Cooking time 45 minutes

Ingredients
2 teaspoons lemon zest
2 teaspoons rosemary, chopped
2 teaspoons red pepper flakes
3 teaspoons salt
3 teaspoons pepper
6 sprigs rosemary
1 (3-pound) whole chicken
Olive oil
⅓ cup Parmesan cheese, finely grated
1-quart chicken stock
Lemon juice to taste

Directions
1. In a mixing bowl, combine the rosemary, pepper flakes, salt, and pepper.
2. Season the chicken with the spice mixture. Stuff 2 rosemary sprigs in the chicken cavity.
3. Add the stock, 2 rosemary sprigs, and chicken (breast side down) to the dry inner cooking pot of the Instant Pot Duo Crisp. Stir with a wooden spatula.
4. Place the pressure lid on top in a lock position.
5. Press PRESSURE. Select HIGH-PRESSURE mode and set the timer to 20 minutes.
6. Press START. After cooking time is over quick release the pressure.
7. Empty the pot and set aside the chicken. Coat the chicken with olive oil.
8. Arrange the air frying basket inside the dry inner pot of the Instant Pot Duo Crisp. Place the chicken inside the basket.

9. Place the air fryer lid on top; press ROAST. Set temperature to 400°F and timer to 25 minutes.
10. Press START. Open lid after half of the time has elapsed, spread the cheese over the chicken, and continue to cook until a food thermometer indicates 160°F.
11. Serve warm with some lemon juice on top.

Nutrition (per serving)
Calories 266, fat 8 g, total carbs 6 g,
Protein 47 g, sodium 1248 mg

Cheesy Chicken Tenders

Serves 6 | Prep. time 5 minutes | Cooking time 12 minutes

Ingredients
1½ pounds chicken tenders
Salt and pepper to taste
½ cup grated Parmesan cheese
1 teaspoon oregano
1 tablespoon paprika
1 teaspoon garlic powder
¼ teaspoon ground thyme (optional)
¼ teaspoon ground mustard (optional)
1 tablespoon unsalted Italian seasoning

Directions
1. In a mixing bowl, combine the Parmesan cheese, oregano, paprika, garlic powder, mustard, thyme, and Italian seasoning.
2. Season the chicken tenders with salt and pepper. Rub the spice mix over them.
3. Arrange the air frying basket inside the dry inner pot of the Instant Pot Duo Crisp. Grease the basket with some vegetable oil or cooking spray.
4. Place the chicken tenders inside the basket.
5. Place the air fryer lid on top; press AIR FRY. Set temperature to 385°F and timer to 12 minutes.
6. Press START. When the Instant P2ot Duo Crisp indicates TURN FOOD, flip the tenders and continue to cook for the remaining time.
7. Serve the tenders with your choice of green salad, mashed potatoes, or roasted carrots/broccoli/cauliflower.

Nutrition (per serving)
Calories 350, fat 19 g, total carbs 3 g,
Protein 23 g, sodium 242 mg

Turkey Skewers

Serves 4 | Prep. time 5–10 minutes | Cooking time 14 minutes

Ingredients
1½ pounds turkey tenderloin, cut into 1-inch pieces
Salt and pepper to taste
1 tablespoon unsalted Italian seasoning
2 teaspoons minced garlic
2 tablespoons olive oil

Directions
1. Season the turkey pieces with salt and pepper to taste.
2. In a mixing bowl, combine the Italian seasoning, garlic, and olive oil.
3. Coat the turkey pieces with the seasoning mix. Add the turkey pieces to a Ziploc bag.
4. Refrigerate for 1–2 hours or overnight to marinate.
5. Thread the turkey pieces onto skewers.
6. Arrange the air frying basket inside the dry inner pot of the Instant Pot Duo Crisp. Grease the basket with some vegetable oil or cooking spray.
7. Place the skewers inside the basket. Cook in batches.
8. Place the air fryer lid on top; press AIR FRY. Set temperature to 350°F and timer to 14 minutes.
9. Press START. When the Instant Pot Duo Crisp indicates TURN FOOD, flip the skewers and continue to cook for the remaining time.
10. Serve warm.

Nutrition (per serving)
Calories 316, fat 10 g, total carbs 1g,
Protein 51 g, sodium 210 mg

Maple Mustard Turkey

Serves 4 | Prep. time 5–10 minutes | Cooking time 35 minutes

Ingredients
2 pounds turkey breasts
½ teaspoon salt
¾ teaspoon pepper
1 teaspoon rosemary, finely chopped
1 teaspoon sage, chopped
1 teaspoon thyme, chopped
¼ cup maple syrup
2 tablespoons Dijon mustard
1 tablespoon butter

Directions
1. Season the turkey breasts with salt and pepper and rub them with rosemary, thyme, and sage.
2. In a mixing bowl, combine the mustard, maple syrup, and butter.
3. Arrange the air frying basket inside the dry inner pot of the Instant Pot Duo Crisp. Grease the basket with some vegetable oil or cooking spray.
4. Place the turkey breasts inside the basket.
5. Place the air fryer lid on top; press AIR FRY. Set temperature to 390°F and timer to 35 minutes.
6. Press START. When the Instant Pot Duo Crisp indicates TURN FOOD, shake the basket and continue to cook for the remaining time.
7. Open the lid and spread the maple mix over the turkey breasts; AIR FRY for 2–3 more minutes.
8. Serve warm.

Nutrition (per serving)
Calories 455, fat 17 g, total carbs 15 g,
Protein 46 g, sodium 495 mg

Chicken Pot Pie

Serves 6 | Prep. time 5–10 minutes | Cooking time 20 minutes

Ingredients
2 tablespoons olive oil
1 pound chicken breast, cut into 1-inch cubes
1 tablespoon garlic powder
1 teaspoon thyme
½ teaspoon pepper
1 cup chicken broth
¾ pound frozen mixed vegetables
4 large potatoes, cut into 1-inch cubes
1 (10-ounce) can cream of chicken soup
1 cup heavy cream
1 pie crust
1 egg
1 tablespoon water

Directions
1. Add the olive oil and chicken to the dry inner pot of the Instant Pot Duo Crisp.
2. Press SAUTE; stir-cook for 4–5 minutes until evenly brown.
3. Mix in the seasoning, broth, and veggies. Pour the soup on top. Do not stir.
4. Place the pressure lid on top in a lock position.
5. Press PRESSURE. Select HIGH-PRESSURE mode and set timer to 10 minutes.
6. Press START. After cooking time is over quick release the pressure.
7. Press SAUTE; stir-cook for 2–3 minutes until the sauce thickens.
8. Place the pie crust on top.
9. Place the air fryer lid on top; press AIR FRY. Set temperature to 400°F and timer to 10 minutes.

10. Press START. When the Instant Pot Duo Crisp indicates TURN FOOD, do nothing.
11. Serve warm.

Nutrition (per serving)
Calories 538, fat 25 g, total carbs 53 g,
Protein 27 g, sodium 544 mg

BEEF, PORK, AND LAMB

Pineapple Jerk Ham

Serves 4 | Prep. time 5–10 minutes | Cooking time 25 minutes

Ingredients
1 cup pineapple juice (divided)
2 tablespoons jerk paste
½ cup brown sugar
¼ cup rum
2 tablespoons lime juice
3 pounds boneless ham, fully cooked and sliced spirally

Directions
1. Add the jerk paste, brown sugar, rum, lime juice, and ½ cup of the pineapple juice to the dry inner pot of the Instant Pot Duo Crisp.
2. Press SAUTE; stir-cook for 2–3 minutes until the mixture thickens.
3. Set the glaze aside; no need to clean the inner pot.
4. Arrange the steam rack inside and arrange the ham over it. Pour in 1 cup of water and the remaining pineapple juice.
5. Place the pressure lid on top in a lock position.
6. Press PRESSURE. Select HIGH-PRESSURE mode and set the timer to 8 minutes.
7. Press START. After cooking time is over natural release the pressure.
8. Drain the liquid and set aside the ham. Glaze it with the reserved glaze.
9. Arrange the air frying basket inside the dry inner pot of the Instant Pot Duo Crisp. Place the ham inside the basket.

10. Place the air fryer lid on top; press BAKE. Set temperature to 400°F and timer to 10–15 minutes.
11. Press START. Cook until the food thermometer indicates 160°F.
12. Serve warm.

Nutrition (per serving)
Calories 590, fat 15 g, total carbs 29 g,
Protein 77 g, sodium 3410 mg

BBQ Pork Ribs

Serves 6 | Prep. time 5–10 minutes | Cooking time 45 minutes

Ingredients
Dry Rub
2 tablespoons smoked paprika
2 tablespoons brown sugar
2 teaspoons pepper
2 tablespoons salt
2 teaspoons chili powder

Ribs
6 pounds pork back ribs
2 cups BBQ sauce
3 cups Coca Cola (or other soda)

Directions
1. In a mixing bowl, combine the dry rub ingredients.
2. Season the ribs with the rub mixture.
3. Add the ribs and cola to the dry inner pot of the Instant Pot Duo Crisp; stir with a wooden spatula.
4. Place the pressure lid on top in a lock position.
5. Press PRESSURE. Select HIGH-PRESSURE mode and set the timer to 15 minutes.
6. Press START. After cooking time is over quick release the pressure.
7. Remove the pork ribs and coat them with BBQ sauce. Clean the inner pot.
8. Arrange the air frying basket inside the dry inner pot of the Instant Pot Duo Crisp. Place the pork ribs inside the basket.
9. Place the air fryer lid on top; press BROIL. Select HIGH-PRESSURE mode and set the timer to 15 minutes.

10. Press START. After cooking time is over quick release the pressure.
11. Serve warm.

Nutrition (per serving)
Calories 261, fat 3 g, total carbs 36 g,
Protein 47 g, sodium 1752 mg

Italian Pasta Delight

Serves 8 | Prep. time 5–10 minutes | Cooking time 25 minutes

Ingredients
1 medium onion
2 tablespoons minced garlic
½–¾ pound Italian sausage
6 ounces pepperoni, sliced
½ teaspoon oregano
½ teaspoon basil
¼ teaspoon pepper
½ teaspoon salt
¼ teaspoon red pepper, crushed
1 cup red wine or chicken stock
2 cups chicken stock
1 (28-ounce) can diced Italian tomatoes, with juice
1 (28-ounce) can tomato puree
1 pound rigatoni or other pasta
½ pound Italian or Mozzarella cheese, shredded

Directions
1. Grease the dry inner pot of the Instant Pot Duo Crisp with some cooking spray. Add the onions, garlic, and sausage.
2. Press SAUTE; stir-cook until sausage is browned.
3. Mix in the spices and half of the pepperoni. Add the red wine and stock. Stir.
4. Mix in the tomatoes and tomato puree. Add the pasta on top; do not stir.
5. Place the pressure lid on top in a lock position.
6. Press PRESSURE. Select HIGH-PRESSURE mode and set timer to 6 minutes.
7. Press START. After cooking time is over quick release the pressure.

8. Add ⅓ of the cheese; stir well. Sprinkle the remaining cheese on top.
9. Place the air fryer lid on top; press AIR FRY. Set temperature to 400°F and timer to 5 minutes.
10. Press START. When the Instant Pot Duo Crisp indicates TURN FOOD, do nothing.
11. Serve warm.

Nutrition (per serving)
Calories 603, fat 33 g, total carbs 42 g,
Protein 29 g, sodium 1218 mg

Korean Lamb Chops

Serves 6 | Prep. time 20 minutes | Cooking time 60 minutes

Ingredients
2 pounds whole lamb
Green onions, chopped, and cilantro to garnish

Sauce
2 tablespoons sugar
1 tablespoon curry powder
2 tablespoons red pepper powder
3 tablespoons soy sauce
3 tablespoons of rice wine
1 teaspoon minced ginger
2 tablespoons minced garlic
2 tablespoons Korean red pepper paste
2 tablespoons ketchup
3/8 cup corn syrup
½ tablespoon sesame oil
½ teaspoon cinnamon powder
1 teaspoon sesame seeds
1 teaspoon pepper
⅓ cup ground Asian pear
⅓ cup onion powder
3 bay leaves
1 cup diced carrots
2 cups diced onions
1 cup diced celery
2 cups water
1 cup red wine

Directions
1. Add all of the sauce ingredients and the whole lamb to the dry inner pot of the Instant Pot Duo Crisp; stir with a wooden spatula.

2. Place the pressure lid on top in a lock position.
3. Press PRESSURE. Select HIGH-PRESSURE mode and set timer to 20 minutes.
4. Press START. After cooking time is over natural release the pressure for about 10–15 minutes.
5. Remove the lamb and set aside to cool.
6. Press SAUTE; stir-cook the sauce until it thickens. Set aside the sauce and clean the inner pot.
7. Cut the lamb into chops.
8. Arrange the air frying basket inside the dry inner pot of the Instant Pot Duo Crisp. Arrange the dehydration rack in the basket. Place the lamb chops on the rack. Cook in batches.
9. Place the air fryer lid on top; press BROIL. Select HIGH-PRESSURE mode and set timer to 5 minutes.
10. Press START. After cooking time is over quick release the pressure.
11. Serve the lamb chops warm with sauce, cilantro, and green onions on top.

Nutrition (per serving)
Calories 669, fat 9 g, total carbs 38 g,
Protein 41 g, sodium 1475 mg

Classic Pot Roast

Serves 6 | Prep. time 10 minutes | Cooking time 70 minutes

Ingredients
2½ pounds chuck roast
1½ teaspoons garlic powder
Salt and pepper to taste
1½ pounds potatoes cut into chunks or baby potatoes
1 pound baby carrots
Optional: fresh herbs (thyme, rosemary, etc.)

Directions
1. Add the chuck roast and water to cover the dry inner pot of the Instant Pot Duo Crisp.
2. Place the pressure lid on top in a lock position.
3. Press PRESSURE. Select HIGH-PRESSURE mode and set the timer to 60 minutes.
4. Press START. After cooking time is over quick release the pressure.
5. Add the carrots and potatoes.
6. Press PRESSURE. Select HIGH-PRESSURE mode and set the timer to 7 minutes.
7. Press START. After cooking time is over natural release the pressure for 5 minutes and then quick-release pressure.
8. Place the air fryer lid on top; press AIR FRY. Set temperature to 450°F and timer to 5 minutes.
9. Press START. When the Instant Pot Duo Crisp indicates TURN FOOD, do nothing. Cook until the top is browned.
10. Serve warm.

Nutrition (per serving)
Calories 456, fat 22 g, total carbs 27 g,
Protein 39 g, sodium 219 mg

Pesto Parmesan Meatballs

Serves 4 | Prep. time 10 minutes | Cooking time 10 minutes

Ingredients
1 pound prepared meatballs, frozen and thawed
1½ cups tomato sauce
¼ cup basil pesto
2 cups shredded mozzarella cheese
½ cup grated Parmesan cheese

Directions
1. Add the tomato sauce and meatballs to the dry inner pot of the Instant Pot Duo Crisp; stir with a wooden spatula.
2. Place the pressure lid on top in a lock position.
3. Press PRESSURE. Select HIGH-PRESSURE mode and set the timer to 5 minutes.
4. Press START. After cooking time is over quick release the pressure.
5. Mix in the pesto and add both kinds of cheese on top.
6. Place the air fryer lid on top; press BROIL. Select HIGH-PRESSURE mode and set the timer to 3–5 minutes.
7. Press START. Cook until cheese is bubbling and golden brown. After cooking time is over quick release the pressure.
8. Serve warm.

Nutrition (per serving)
Calories 660 fat 49 g, total carbs 19 g,
Protein 40 g, sodium 1580 mg

Peach Pork Chops

Serves 2–3 | Prep. time 5–10 minutes | Cooking time 12 minutes

Ingredients
1 tablespoon Dijon mustard
1 tablespoon balsamic vinegar
1 pound boneless pork chops
1 teaspoon olive oil
Salt and pepper to taste

Peaches
1 teaspoon balsamic vinegar
2 medium peaches, sliced

Directions
1. In a mixing bowl, combine the vinegar and mustard.
2. Pat the pork chops dry and coats them with olive oil. Season with salt and pepper to taste.
3. Coat the pork chops with the mustard mixture.
4. Arrange the air frying basket inside the dry inner pot of the Instant Pot Duo Crisp. Grease the basket with some vegetable oil or cooking spray.
5. Place the pork chops inside the basket.
6. Place the air fryer lid on top; press AIR FRY. Set temperature to 400°F and timer to 12 minutes.
7. Press START. When the Instant Pot Duo Crisp indicates TURN FOOD, flip the pork chops and continue to cook for the remaining time.
8. In a mixing bowl, combine the peaches and vinegar.
9. Arrange the air frying basket inside the dry inner pot of the Instant Pot Duo Crisp. Grease the basket with some vegetable oil or cooking spray.
10. Place the peach mixture inside the basket.
11. Place the air fryer lid on top; press AIR FRY. Set temperature to 400°F and timer to 2 minutes.

12. Press START. When the Instant Pot Duo Crisp indicates TURN FOOD, do nothing. Cook until peaches are softened.
13. Serve the pork chops with the peach mixture on top.

Nutrition (per serving)
Calories 431, fat 23 g, total carbs 17 g,
Protein 42 g, sodium 267 mg

Shepherd's Pie

Serves 6 | Prep. time 10–15 minutes | Cooking time 45 minutes

Ingredients
2 tablespoons butter
½ pound mushrooms, sliced
½ teaspoon salt
½ teaspoon pepper
1 stalk celery, diced
1 carrot, diced
1 onion, diced
1 tablespoon rosemary, finely chopped
2 cloves garlic, minced
2 tablespoons tomato paste
1½ pounds ground beef
1 tablespoon Worcestershire sauce
1½ cups low-sodium beef broth
1 tablespoon Dijon mustard
3 tablespoons all-purpose flour
4 cups hash browns, shredded
1 cup shredded aged cheddar cheese
⅓ cup Parmesan cheese, grated
2 tablespoons parsley, finely

Directions
1. Add the butter, mushrooms, ¼ teaspoon of pepper, and ¼ teaspoon of salt to the dry inner pot of the Instant Pot Duo Crisp.
2. Press SAUTE; stir-cook for 3–5 minutes until softened and light brown.
3. Mix in the remaining salt and pepper along with the celery, carrot, onion, rosemary, and garlic; stir-cook for 2–3 minutes until softened.
4. Mix in the beef and cook for 3–5 minutes until evenly brown.

5. Mix in tomato paste and cook for 1 minute.
6. Add the Worcestershire sauce, broth, and mustard. Stir gently.
7. Place the pressure lid on top in a lock position.
8. Press PRESSURE. Select HIGH-PRESSURE mode and set timer to 4 minutes.
9. Press START. After cooking time is over quick release the pressure.
10. In a bowl, mix 2 tablespoons of water with the flour. Mix into the beef mixture.
11. Press SAUTE; stir-cook for 2–3 minutes until the sauce thickens.
12. Add the hash browns and sprinkle both kinds of cheese on top.
13. Place the air fryer lid on top; press ROAST. Set temperature to 400°F and timer to 25–35 minutes.
14. Press START. Cook until cheese is bubbling and golden brown.
15. Serve warm with parsley on top.

Nutrition (per serving)
Calories 550, fat 30 g, total carbs 35 g,
Protein 34 g, sodium 790 mg

Gammon Steak Rice

Serves 4 | Prep. time 5–10 minutes | Cooking time 15–18 minutes

Ingredients
1 teaspoon olive oil
1 onion, chopped
1 medium carrot, chopped
3 cloves garlic, chopped
½ stalk celery, finely chopped
Dash of wine
10–11 ounces Arborio rice
3½ cups gammon steak stock
3½ ounce Gammon steak, diced
3 ounces aged cheddar cheese

Directions
1. Add the olive oil, carrots, garlic, celery, and onion to the dry inner pot of the Instant Pot Duo Crisp.
2. Press SAUTE; stir-cook for a few minutes until the veggies are softened.
3. Mix in the wine and rice. Stir and cook for 1–2 minutes.
4. Pour in the stock and stir again.
5. Place the pressure lid on top in a lock position.
6. Press PRESSURE. Select HIGH- PRESSURE mode and set the timer to 5 minutes.
7. Press START. After cooking time is over quick release the pressure.
8. Mix in the ham. Season with salt to taste, if desired. Sprinkle the cheese on top.
9. Place the air fryer lid on top; press BROIL. Select HIGH-PRESSURE mode and set the timer to 6 minutes.

10. Press START; cook until ham is cooked to satisfaction. After cooking time is over quick release the pressure. Cook for 2–3 minutes more, if needed.
11. Serve warm.

Nutrition (per serving)
Calories 298, fat 9 g, total carbs 42 g,
Protein 9 g, sodium 177 mg

Stuffed Peppers

Serves 4 | Prep. time 5–10 minutes | Cooking time 25 minutes

Ingredients
2 (2-ounce) chipotle peppers in adobo + sauce
2 tablespoons lime juice
1½ cups beer
5 cloves garlic
1–2 handfuls cilantro
1 teaspoon salt
1 pound 93% lean ground beef
4 large bell peppers
½ teaspoon ground cumin
3 ounces pepper jack cheese, shredded

Directions
1. In a blender or food processor, blend the chipotle peppers, lime juice, beer, garlic, cilantro, and salt until smooth.
2. Grease the dry inner pot of the Instant Pot Duo Crisp with some cooking spray. Add the ground beef.
3. Press SAUTE; stir-cook until evenly brown.
4. Mix in the beer mixture and stir-cook for 8–10 minutes more. Set aside.
5. Cut the tops off of the peppers; remove the seeds. Stuff with the beef mixture.
6. Arrange the air frying basket inside the dry inner pot of the Instant Pot Duo Crisp. Grease the basket with some vegetable oil or cooking spray.
7. Place the peppers inside the basket.
8. Place the air fryer lid on top; press AIR FRY. Set temperature to 375°F and timer to 12 minutes.
9. Press START. When the Instant Pot Duo Crisp indicates TURN FOOD, do nothing.

10. Add the cheese on top of the peppers; AIR FRY for 6–8 minutes more.
11. Serve warm.

Nutrition (per serving)
Calories 365, fat 19 g, total carbs 13 g,
Protein 31 g, sodium 560 mg

Sausage and Onions

Serves 4 | Prep. time 5–10 minutes | Cooking time 30 minutes

Ingredients
1¼ pounds smoked sausage, sliced
2 onions, diced
2 tablespoons olive oil
Salt and pepper to taste

Directions
1. Grease the dry inner pot of the Instant Pot Duo Crisp with some cooking spray. Add the onions, salt, and pepper.
2. Press SAUTE; stir-cook until softened and translucent. Set onions aside.
3. Arrange the air frying basket inside the dry inner pot of the Instant Pot Duo Crisp. Grease the basket with some vegetable oil or cooking spray.
4. Place the onions and sausage inside the basket.
5. Place the air fryer lid on top; press AIR FRY. Set temperature to 400°F and timer to 25–30 minutes.
6. Press START. When the Instant Pot Duo Crisp indicates TURN FOOD, stir a bit and continue to cook for the remaining time.
7. Serve warm.

Nutrition (per serving)
Calories 754, fat 69 g, total carbs 5 g,
Protein 28 g, sodium 1925 mg

FISH AND SEAFOOD

Mayonnaise Salmon with Dill Sauce

Serves 4 | Prep. time 5–10 minutes | Cooking time 7 minutes

Ingredients
4 salmon fillets
2 tablespoons olive oil
Salt and pepper to taste
½ teaspoon paprika (optional)
⅓ cup sour cream
⅓ cup mayonnaise
Zest and juice of 1 lemon
1 teaspoon garlic
½ teaspoon English-style mustard
2–3 tablespoons fresh dill or 2 teaspoons dried dill

Directions
1. Coat the fish fillets with olive oil and season with pepper, paprika, and salt.
2. Arrange the air frying basket inside the dry inner pot of the Instant Pot Duo Crisp. Grease the basket with some vegetable oil or cooking spray.
3. Place the fish fillets inside the basket.
4. Place the air fryer lid on top; press AIR FRY. Set temperature to 390°F and timer to 8 minutes.
5. Press START. When the Instant Pot Duo Crisp indicates TURN FOOD, do nothing. Cook until salmon is cooked through. Cook for a couple of minutes more, if needed.
6. In a mixing bowl, combine the sour cream, mayo, lemon juice, garlic, mustard, and dill.
7. Serve the salmon fillets with dill sauce on top.

Nutrition (per serving)
Calories 702, fat 53 g, total carbs 2 g,
Protein 51 g, sodium 342 mg

Cod with Mustard Sauce

Serves 2 | Prep. time 5–10 minutes | Cooking time 10 minutes

Ingredients
1 tablespoon lemon juice
½ teaspoon pepper
½ teaspoon salt
2 tablespoons olive oil
1 pound cod fillets

Sauce
3 tablespoons ground mustard
1 tablespoon butter
½ cup heavy cream
½ teaspoon salt

Directions
1. Coat the cod fillets with olive oil; season with salt and pepper. Drizzle the lemon juice on top.
2. Arrange the air frying basket inside the dry inner pot of the Instant Pot Duo Crisp. Grease the basket with some vegetable oil or cooking spray.
3. Place the fillets inside the basket.
4. Place the air fryer lid on top; press AIR FRY. Set temperature to 350°F and timer to 10 minutes.
5. Press START. When the Instant Pot Duo Crisp indicates TURN FOOD, flip the fillets and continue to cook for the remaining time.
6. Transfer the fish fillets to a serving plate.
7. Remove the basket. Add the butter, mustard, heavy cream, and salt to the inner cooking pot.
8. Press SAUTE; stir-cook for 3–4 minutes.
9. Pour the warm sauce over fish fillets before serving.

Nutrition (per serving)
Calories 498, fat 29 g, total carbs 19 g, Protein 30 g, sodium 1203 mg

Fish Tacos

Serves 4 | Prep. time 15–20 minutes | Cooking time 10 minutes

Ingredients
½ cup cornmeal
½ cup breadcrumbs
1 pound cod, haddock or tilapia, sliced into 2-inch strips
1 tablespoon taco seasoning
¼ cup all-purpose flour
1 egg, lightly beaten
1 tablespoon olive oil
4 teaspoons canola oil
½ cup sour cream
⅓ cup cilantro, finely chopped
1 tablespoon lime juice
1 clove garlic, minced
¼ teaspoon salt
1 tablespoon minced jalapeño pepper
¼ teaspoon pepper
¼ teaspoon oregano
¼ teaspoon cumin
8 corn tortillas, warmed
1 cup shredded cabbage
4 radishes, thinly sliced
Lime wedges to serve

Directions
1. In a mixing bowl, combine the cornmeal and breadcrumbs.
2. Coat the fish strips with taco seasoning.
3. Beat the egg in one bowl and add the flour to another bowl.
4. Coat the fish strips with egg and then with flour. Lastly, coat with the crumb mixture.

5. Arrange the air frying basket inside the dry inner pot of the Instant Pot Duo Crisp. Grease the basket with some vegetable oil or cooking spray.
6. Cook in two batches. Place half of the fish strips inside the basket. Drizzle with half of the olive oil.
7. Place the air fryer lid on top; press AIR FRY. Set temperature to 400°F and timer to 4–5 minutes.
8. Press START. When the Instant Pot Duo Crisp indicates TURN FOOD, shake the basket gently and continue to cook for the remaining time until fish strips are golden brown.
9. In a mixing bowl, combine the canola oil, sour cream, cilantro, lime juice, garlic, salt, jalapeño, black, pepper, oregano, and cumin.
10. Arrange the tortillas and add the fish strips, cabbage, sour cream mixture, and radishes.
11. Serve with lime wedges.

Nutrition (per serving)
Calories 490, fat 17 g, total carbs 56 g,
Protein 29 g, sodium 570 mg

Coconut Shrimp Meal

Serves 46 | Prep. time 5–10 minutes | Cooking time 6 minutes

Ingredients
2 large eggs
¼ cup honey
1 serrano chili, thinly sliced
¼ cup lime juice
½ cup all-purpose flour
½ teaspoon pepper
½ teaspoon salt
3 cups unsweetened flaked coconut
3 cups panko breadcrumbs
2 teaspoons chopped cilantro
¾ pound raw shrimp, peeled and deveined

Directions
1. In a mixing bowl, beat the eggs. Mix in the honey, serrano chili, and lime juice.
2. In another mixing bowl, combine the flour, salt, and pepper.
3. In another mixing bowl, combine the breadcrumbs and flaked coconut.
4. Coat the shrimp with egg mixture, then with the flour mixture, and then with the crumbs.
5. Arrange the air frying basket inside the dry inner pot of the Instant Pot Duo Crisp. Line it with parchment paper.
6. Place the coated shrimp inside the basket and spray them with some cooking spray.
7. Place the air fryer lid on top; press AIR FRY. Set temperature to 400°F and timer to 6 minutes.
8. Press START. When the Instant Pot Duo Crisp indicates TURN FOOD, shake the basket gently and

continue to cook for the remaining time until golden brown.
9. Serve warm.

Nutrition *(per serving)*
Calories 258, fat 9 g, total carbs 31 g,
Protein 14 g, sodium 366 mg

Seasoned Super Salmon

Serves 2 | Prep. time 5 minutes | Cooking time 7 minutes

Ingredients
2 (6-ounce) salmon fillets
2 teaspoons olive oil
1 teaspoon garlic powder
1 teaspoon onion powder
1 teaspoon paprika
Salt and pepper
2 green onions, thinly sliced
4 teaspoons toasted sesame seeds

Directions
1. In a mixing bowl, combine the garlic powder, onion powder, paprika, salt, and pepper.
2. Coat the salmon fillets with olive oil.
3. Arrange the air frying basket inside the dry inner pot of the Instant Pot Duo Crisp. Grease the basket with some vegetable oil or cooking spray.
4. Place the salmon fillets inside the basket.
5. Place the air fryer lid on top; press AIR FRY. Set temperature to 400°F and timer to 8 minutes.
6. Press START. When the Instant Pot Duo Crisp indicates TURN FOOD, do nothing.
7. Serve warm.

Nutrition (per serving)
Calories 53, fat 5 g, total carbs 3 g,
Protein 1 g, sodium 150 mg

MEATLESS

Mac and Cheese

Serves 4 | Prep. time 5–10 minutes | Cooking time 10 minutes

Ingredients
½ cup butter (divided)
2 cups chicken stock
2½ cups macaroni
¼ teaspoon garlic powder
1¼ cups heavy cream
2⅔ cups shredded cheese (sharp cheddar, Mexican blend, pepper jack, etc.)
⅓ cup shredded Parmesan cheese
1 sleeve Ritz crackers
Salt and pepper to taste

Directions
1. Add the stock, pasta, garlic powder, heavy cream, and ¼ cup of the butter to the dry inner pot of the Instant Pot Duo Crisp; stir with a wooden spatula.
2. Place the pressure lid on top in a lock position.
3. Press PRESSURE. Select HIGH-PRESSURE mode and set the timer to 4 minutes.
4. Press START. After cooking time is over quick release the pressure.
5. In a mixing bowl, combine the remaining butter and Ritz crackers.
6. Mix 2 cups of the shredded cheese into the pot until it melts completely.
7. Spread the remaining cheese, Parmesan, and cracker mix on top.

8. Place the air fryer lid on top; press AIR FRY. Set temperature to 400°F and timer to 5 minutes.
9. Press START. When the Instant Pot Duo Crisp indicates TURN FOOD, do nothing. Cook until the mixture is evenly brown.
10. Serve warm.

Nutrition (per serving)
Calories 675, fat 56 g, total carbs 22 g,
Protein 22 g, sodium 765 mg

Rosemary Roast Potatoes

Serves 4–6 | Prep. time 10 minutes | Cooking time 20 minutes

Ingredients
1 tablespoon rosemary leaves
1½ teaspoons salt
1 teaspoon black or pink peppercorns
1 (2–3 pound) eye of round roast
½–1 tablespoon olive oil
1–2 tablespoons unsalted butter
Honey to taste
Roast potatoes, sliced into rounds

Horseradish Cream
⅓ cup sour cream
1½ tablespoons prepared horseradish
¼ teaspoon salt
1 tablespoon honey

Directions
1. Using a mortar and pestle, make a paste from the rosemary, peppercorns, and salt.
2. Coat the roast with olive oil. Rub the paste over the roast.
3. Arrange the air frying basket inside the dry inner pot of the Instant Pot Duo Crisp. Grease the basket with some vegetable oil or cooking spray.
4. Place the roast inside the basket.
5. Place the air fryer lid on top; press AIR FRY. Set temperature to 325°F and timer to 16–18 minutes.
6. Press START. When the Instant Pot Duo Crisp indicates TURN FOOD, flip the roast and continue to cook for the remaining time until a food thermometer indicates 130–135°F.

7. Set aside on a cutting board; top with the butter and drizzle with honey.
8. Cover with aluminum foil and set aside for 15–20 minutes.
9. In a mixing bowl, combine the cream ingredients.
10. Slice the roast into thin slices and serve with potatoes and the prepared cream.

Tofu Coconut Curry

Serves 2–3 | Prep. time 10–15 minutes | Cooking time 30 minutes

Ingredients
1 pound extra-firm tofu, drained and cut into ½-inch cubes
1 clove garlic, minced
2 tablespoons soy sauce
2 tablespoons toasted sesame oil
1 tablespoon olive oil
1 small onion, finely diced
1 red pepper, chopped
2 yellow squash, cut into half-moons
1 head broccoli, cut into florets
2 tablespoons red curry paste
2 teaspoons salt
1 (15-ounce) can coconut milk
2 cups cooked rice
Chopped

Directions
1. In a Ziploc bag, combine the tofu cubes, garlic, soy sauce, and sesame oil. Shake to mix well. Set aside for 15 minutes.
2. Add the olive oil and onions to the dry inner pot of the Instant Pot Duo Crisp.
3. Press SAUTE; stir-cook for 3–4 minutes until softened and translucent.
4. Add the red pepper, squash, broccoli, curry paste, and salt. Stir-cook for 2–3 minutes.
5. Mix in the coconut milk.
6. Place the pressure lid on top in a lock position.
7. Press PRESSURE. Select HIGH-PRESSURE mode and set timer to 10 minutes.
8. Press START. After cooking time is over quick release the pressure.

9. Set aside the cooked mixture and clean the inner pot.
10. Drain the marinade from the tofu.
11. Arrange the air frying basket inside the dry inner pot of the Instant Pot Duo Crisp. Add half of the tofu to the basket.
12. Arrange the broiling tray and place the remaining tofu over it.
13. Place the air fryer lid on top; press AIR FRY. Set temperature to 375°F and timer to 15 minutes.
14. Press START. When the Instant Pot Duo Crisp indicates TURN FOOD, shake the basket and continue to cook for the remaining time.
15. Add the cooked rice to serving plates; serve warm topped with the curried veggies and tofu.

French Onion Soup

Serves 5 | Prep. time 5–10 minutes | Cooking time 45 minutes

Ingredients
3 tablespoons butter
1 tablespoon olive oil
2 large white onions cut into ¼ inch slices
1 sweet onion, cut into ¼ inch slices
2 cloves garlic, minced
1 tablespoon tomato paste
½ cup + 2 tablespoons red wine
1 tablespoon soy sauce
4¾ cups beef stock
1 tablespoon Worcestershire sauce
Salt and pepper to taste
2 cups 1-inch cubes of French bread
2 cups shredded mozzarella and Gruyere cheese

<u>Herb Mix</u>
1 bay leaf
1 sprig thyme
1 sprig fresh rosemary
3 sprigs flat-leaf parsley
5 peppercorns

Directions
1. Add the herb mix ingredients to a cloth bag; tie with a string.
2. Add the olive oil, butter, salt, garlic, and onions to the dry inner pot of the Instant Pot Duo Crisp.
3. Press SAUTE; stir-cook for 15–20 minutes until the onions are caramelized.
4. Pour in the red wine and tomato paste. Cook for 3 minutes.

5. Add the soy sauce, beef stock, Worcestershire sauce, and herb bag. Mix well.
6. Season with salt and pepper.
7. Place the pressure lid on top in a lock position.
8. Press PRESSURE. Select HIGH-PRESSURE mode and set timer to 10 minutes.
9. Press START. After cooking time is over quick release the pressure.
10. Season with salt and pepper to taste.
11. Top with the bread cubes and shredded cheese.
12. Place the air fryer lid on top; press BROIL. Select HIGH-PRESSURE mode and set the timer to 7 minutes.
13. Press START. After cooking time is over quick release the pressure.
14. Serve warm.

Jalapeño Mac and Cheese

Serves 4 | Prep. time 10–15 minutes | Cooking time 15 minutes

Ingredients
2 jalapeño peppers, seeded
¼ cup butter
3 cloves garlic, minced
1 onion, diced
2 teaspoons chili powder
1½ teaspoons ground cumin
¼ teaspoon cayenne pepper
1 pound elbow macaroni
2 teaspoons salt
1½ cups shredded aged cheddar
1 cup heavy cream
1 cup sour cream
8 ounces plain cream cheese, cubed
2 tablespoons Dijon mustard
⅓ cup grated Parmesan cheese
⅓ cup panko breadcrumbs

Directions
1. Partially cook the pasta (around 2 minutes less than specified on the package); drain and set aside.
2. Thinly slice 1 jalapeño and dice the other one.
3. Add the garlic, onion, diced jalapeño, chili powder, cumin, cayenne pepper, and half of the butter to the dry inner pot of the Instant Pot Duo Crisp.
4. Press SAUTE; stir-cook for 2–3 minutes until softened.
5. Pour in 1 quart of water. Add the salt and pasta.
6. Place the pressure lid on top in a lock position.
7. Press PRESSURE. Select HIGH-PRESSURE mode and set timer to 4 minutes.

8. Press START. After cooking time is over quick release the pressure.
9. Stir in the cheddar, heavy cream, sour cream, cream cheese, and mustard.
10. In a mixing bowl, combine the reserved butter, Parmesan, and breadcrumbs. Add to the pasta mix.
11. Add the sliced jalapeño.
12. Place the air fryer lid on top; press ROAST. Set temperature to 400°F and timer to 5 minutes.
13. Press START. Cook until the top is golden brown and bubbling.
14. Serve warm.

Nutrition (per serving)
Calories 1260, fat 80 g, total carbs 102 g,
Protein 37 g, sodium 2210 mg

Macaroni Veggie Delight

Serves 4 | Prep. time 5–10 minutes | Cooking time 6 minutes

Ingredients
1 teaspoon olive oil
1 small zucchini, diced
1 small red pepper, diced
½ piece eggplant, diced
14 ounces chopped tomatoes
2 cups vegetable stock
10½ ounces macaroni pasta

Directions
1. Add the olive oil and veggies to the dry inner pot of the Instant Pot Duo Crisp.
2. Press SAUTE; stir-cook for 4–5 minutes until softened.
3. Stir in the stock and tomatoes.
4. Mix in the pasta.
5. Place the pressure lid on top in a lock position.
6. Press PRESSURE. Select HIGH-PRESSURE mode and set timer to 2 minutes.
7. Press START. After cooking time is over quick release the pressure.
8. Sprinkle the cheese on top.
9. Place the air fryer lid on top; press BROIL. Select HIGH-PRESSURE mode and set timer to 4 minutes.
10. Press START. After cooking time is over quick release the pressure.
11. Serve warm.

SIDES

Mystery Chicken Wings

Serves 4 | Prep. time 5–10 minutes | Cooking time 60 minutes

Ingredients
2 pounds chicken wings split
½ teaspoon salt
½ teaspoon pepper
¼ cup all-purpose flour
2 tablespoons canola oil
2 tablespoons sriracha hot sauce
¼ cup maple syrup
2 tablespoons white miso paste
2 cloves garlic, minced

Directions
1. Season the wings with salt and pepper.
2. Add the flour and chicken wings to a bowl. Toss to coat well.
3. Arrange the air frying basket inside the dry inner pot of the Instant Pot Duo Crisp. Grease the basket with some vegetable oil or cooking spray.
4. Place the chicken wings inside the basket. Drizzle with canola oil. If needed, cook in batches.
5. Place the air fryer lid on top; press AIR FRY. Set temperature to 400°F and timer to 20 minutes.
6. Press START. When the Instant Pot Duo Crisp indicates TURN FOOD, flip the chicken wings and continue to cook for the remaining time until crispy and golden brown.
7. In a mixing bowl, combine the hot sauce, maple syrup, miso, and garlic.

8. Add the chicken wings and coat well; serve and enjoy.

Nutrition (per serving)
Calories 390, fat 23 g, total carbs 24 g,
Protein 23 g, sodium 830 mg

Corn on the Cob

*Serves 3 | Prep. time 5–10 minutes |
Cooking time 12 minutes*

Ingredients
3 ears corn on the cob, shucked and cleaned
¼ teaspoon chili powder
2 tablespoons unsalted butter, softened
½ teaspoon lime juice
Parmesan cheese or goat cheese, shredded
Paprika

Directions
1. Cut the corn in halves if too large to fit into the basket.
2. Arrange the air frying basket inside the dry inner pot of the Instant Pot Duo Crisp. Grease the basket with some vegetable oil or cooking spray.
3. Place the corn inside the basket.
4. Place the air fryer lid on top; press AIR FRY. Set temperature to 400°F and timer to 12 minutes.
5. Press START. When the Instant Pot Duo Crisp indicates TURN FOOD, flip the corn and continue to cook for the remaining time until light brown and tender.
6. In a mixing bowl, combine the chili powder, butter, and lime juice.
7. Top the cooked corn cobs with the shredded cheese and serve warm with butter dip.

Nutrition (per serving)
Calories 170, fat 9 g, total carbs 22 g,
Protein 4 g, sodium 261 mg

Honeyed Brussels Sprouts

Serves 2–4 | Prep. time 5–10 minutes | Cooking time 20 minutes

Ingredients
1 tablespoon olive oil
1 pound Brussels sprouts, trimmed and halved
¼ teaspoon red pepper flakes
Salt to taste
2 tablespoons honey
Juice of 1 lime

Directions
1. In a mixing bowl, combine the olive oil, Brussels sprouts, red pepper flakes, and salt.
2. Arrange the air frying basket inside the dry inner pot of the Instant Pot Duo Crisp. Grease the basket with some vegetable oil or cooking spray.
3. Place the sprouts inside the basket.
4. Place the air fryer lid on top; press AIR FRY. Set temperature to 350°F and timer to 20 minutes.
5. Press START. When the Instant Pot Duo Crisp indicates TURN FOOD, shake the basket and continue to cook for the remaining time.
6. In a mixing bowl, combine the honey, lime juice, and a pinch of salt.
7. Add the sprouts and toss to coat well. Serve warm.

Pizza Dip

Serves 6 | Prep. time 10 minutes | Cooking time 10 minutes

Ingredients
½ cup mayonnaise
½ cup pizza sauce
8 ounces plain cream cheese
1 teaspoon Italian herb seasoning
2 cloves garlic, minced
¼ teaspoon salt and pepper
4 ounces mozzarella cheese, cubed
1 cup shredded mozzarella cheese
½ cup grated Parmesan cheese
8 thin pepperoni slices
2 tablespoons basil, thinly sliced
Assorted crackers or bread to serve

Directions
1. In a mixing bowl, combine the mayonnaise, pizza sauce, cream cheese, Italian herb seasoning, garlic, salt, and pepper.
2. Mix in the mozzarella cubes, half of the shredded mozzarella, and half of the Parmesan.
3. Coat a 6–7-inch round baking pan with olive oil.
4. Add the cheese mixture and top with the remaining mozzarella and Parmesan.
5. Top with the pepperoni.
6. Arrange the air frying basket inside the dry inner pot of the Instant Pot Duo Crisp. Place the baking dish inside the basket.
7. Place the air fryer lid on top; press BAKE. Set temperature to 400°F and timer to 10–15 minutes.
8. Press START. Bake until dip is bubbly and golden brown.
9. Add the basil on top and serve warm with crackers and/or bread.

Nutrition (per serving)
Calories 430, fat 39 g, total carbs 5g,
Protein 17 g, sodium 910 mg

Baked Beans with Nachos

Serves 6 | Prep. time 5–10 minutes | Cooking time 45 minutes

Ingredients
2 tablespoons olive oil
1½ teaspoons minced or thinly sliced garlic
3 tablespoons tomato paste
1⅓ cups cannellini or great northern beans washed and dried
Salt and pepper to taste
1⅓ cups mozzarella, coarsely grated
Nacho chips or toasted bread to serve

Directions
1. Add the beans and 1 quart of water to the dry inner pot of the Instant Pot Duo Crisp; stir with a wooden spatula.
2. Place the pressure lid on top in a lock position.
3. Press PRESSURE. Select HIGH-PRESSURE mode and set timer to 25 minutes.
4. Press START. After cooking time is over quick release the pressure.
5. Drain the beans and set them aside. Empty the inner pot.
6. Add the olive oil and garlic.
7. Press SAUTE; stir-cook for about 30–60 seconds until fragrant.
8. Mix in tomato paste and cook for 30 seconds.
9. Add the beans, salt, and pepper; stir. Add more water as needed.
10. Sprinkle the mozzarella on top.
11. Place the air fryer lid on top; press BROIL. Select HIGH-PRESSURE mode and set the timer to 7 minutes.

12. Press START. After cooking time is over quick release the pressure.
13. Serve with nacho chips or toasted bread.

Roasted Parsnips

Serves 4–6 | Prep.time 5–10 minutes | Cooking time 20 minutes

Ingredients
2 pounds parsnips
2 cups cold water
1 tablespoon olive oil
Dipping sauce of your choice

Directions
1. Rinse the parsnips and slice them lengthwise into 2 or 4 strips.
2. Pour 2 cups of water into the dry inner pot of the Instant Pot Duo Crisp. Arrange the steam rack and place the parsnips strips over it.
3. Place the pressure lid on top in a lock position.
4. Press STEAM. Set timer to 5 minutes.
5. Press START. After cooking time is over quick release the pressure.
6. Drain the water and transfer the parsnip strips to a bowl. Coat them with olive oil.
7. Arrange the air frying basket inside the dry inner pot of the Instant Pot Duo Crisp. Place the parsnip strips inside the basket.
8. Place the air fryer lid on top; press ROAST. Set temperature to 400°F and timer to 20 minutes.
9. Press START. After half of the cooking time has elapsed, flip the strips, and continue to cook.
10. Serve warm with your choice of dipping sauce.

Pancetta Brussels Sprouts

Serves 4 | Prep. time 5–10 minutes | Cooking time 18 minutes

Ingredients
1 pound Brussels sprouts, trimmed and halved
4 ounces pancetta, chopped
Olive oil as needed
1 tablespoon balsamic vinegar glaze

Directions
1. In a mixing bowl, combine the Brussels sprouts, pancetta, and olive oil.
2. Arrange the air frying basket inside the dry inner pot of the Instant Pot Duo Crisp. Grease the basket with some vegetable oil or cooking spray.
3. Place the sprouts inside the basket.
4. Place the air fryer lid on top; press AIR FRY. Set temperature to 350°F and timer to 18 minutes.
5. Press START. When the Instant Pot Duo Crisp indicates TURN FOOD, shake the basket and continue to cook for the remaining time. Air fry for 2 minutes more if you want crispier sprouts.
6. Transfer the sprouts to a bowl and add the vinegar glaze; toss to mix well.
7. Serve warm.

Nutrition (per serving)
Calories 220 fat 16 g, total carbs 16 g,
Protein 6 g, sodium 35 mg

DESSERTS

S'mores Delight

Serves 8 | Prep. time 10–15 minutes | Cooking time 30 minutes

Ingredients
1 cup all-purpose flour
1 teaspoon baking powder
½ teaspoon salt
1 cup brown sugar
½ cup butter, melted
1 egg
1 teaspoon vanilla extract
⅔ cup pecans, chopped (divided)
½ cup dark chocolate chunks
4 square graham crackers, torn into pieces
½ cup mini marshmallows
Pinch of flaked sea salt
¼ cup dulce de leche

Directions
1. Line a 6–7-inch round baking pan with parchment paper.
2. In a mixing bowl, combine the flour, baking powder, and ½ teaspoon of salt. Add ½ cup of the pecans.
3. In a mixing bowl, beat butter and sugar until the sugar dissolves. Mix in the egg and vanilla.
4. Combine the two mixtures and mix well.
5. Pour the batter into the pan.
6. Arrange the steam rack in the dry inner pot of the Instant Pot Duo Crisp and place the pan over it.
7. Place the air fryer lid on top; press BAKE. Set temperature to 350°F and timer to 25 minutes.

8. Press START. Bake until an inserted toothpick comes out clean.
9. Top with the remaining pecans, chocolate, graham crackers, marshmallows, and sea salt.
10. Pour the dulce de leche on top.
11. Place the air fryer lid on top; press BROIL. Select HIGH-PRESSURE mode and set timer to 3–5 minutes.
12. Press START. After cooking time is over quick release the pressure.
13. Serve warm.

Nutrition (per serving)
Calories 400, fat 23 g, total carbs 48 g,
Protein 5 g, sodium 350 mg

Cinnamon Apple Cake

Serves 6 | Prep. time 15–20 minutes | Cooking time 40 minutes

Ingredients
Cake
1 cup all-purpose flour
¼ cup almond flour
¼ cup fine cornmeal
1 teaspoon baking powder
½ teaspoon baking soda
¼ teaspoon salt
¾ cup of sugar
2 eggs
2 tablespoons honey
¾ cup plain 2% yogurt
½ cup olive oil
2 teaspoons lemon zest
1 teaspoon vanilla extract

Apples
2 tablespoons butter
½ cup sugar
2 tablespoons corn syrup
¼ teaspoon ground cinnamon
4 peeled and cored apples, sliced

Directions
1. In a mixing bowl, combine the flour, almond flour, cornmeal, salt, baking powder, and baking soda.
2. In another mixing bowl, beat the eggs. Mix in the honey and sugar.
3. Add the olive oil, lemon zest, yogurt, and vanilla and beat until mixed well.
4. Combine the two mixtures and mix well.

5. Line an 8-inch cake pan with parchment paper. Pour in the batter.
6. Arrange the steam rack in the dry inner pot of the Instant Pot Duo Crisp and place the cake pan over it.
7. Place the air fryer lid on top; press BAKE. Set temperature to 350°F and timer to 25–30 minutes.
8. Press START. Bake until an inserted toothpick comes out clean. Set the cake aside.
9. Add the butter, corn syrup, apples, sugar, and cinnamon to the inner pot.
10. Press SAUTE; stir-cook for 8–10 minutes until caramelized.
11. Slice the cake into 6 pieces and top with the caramelized apples.

Nutrition (per serving)
Calories 610, fat 27 g, total carbs 90 g,
Protein 7 g, sodium 340 mg

RECIPE INDEX

APPETIZERS AND SNACKS   **5**
    Crispy Sausage Bites   5
    French Fries   7
    Cauliflower Crisp Bites   8
    Prosciutto Wrapped Dates   9
    Fried Cheesy Pickles   10
    Falafel   11
    Chicken Kebabs   13

CHICKEN AND POULTRY   **15**
    Chicken Broccoli Casserole   15
    Chicken Poutine   17
    Orange Roast Chicken   19
    BBQ Drumsticks   21
    Seasoned Whole Chicken   23
    Red Hot Chicken Wings   25
    Turkey Meatloaf   27
    Parmesan Chicken Roast   29
    Cheesy Chicken Tenders   31
    Turkey Skewers   33
    Maple Mustard Turkey   34
    Chicken Pot Pie   35

BEEF, PORK, AND LAMB   **37**
    Pineapple Jerk Ham   37
    BBQ Pork Ribs   39
    Italian Pasta Delight   41
    Korean Lamb Chops   43
    Classic Pot Roast   45
    Pesto Parmesan Meatballs   46
    Peach Pork Chops   47
    Shepherd's Pie   49
    Gammon Steak Rice   51
    Stuffed Peppers   53
    Sausage and Onions   55

FISH AND SEAFOOD   57
    Mayonnaise Salmon with Dill Sauce   57
    Cod with Mustard Sauce   59
    Fish Tacos   61
    Coconut Shrimp Meal   63
    Seasoned Super Salmon   65

MEATLESS   67
    Mac and Cheese   67
    Rosemary Roast Potatoes   69
    Tofu Coconut Curry   71
    French Onion Soup   73
    Jalapeño Mac and Cheese   75
    Macaroni Veggie Delight   77

SIDES   79
    Mystery Chicken Wings   79
    Corn on the Cob   81
    Honeyed Brussels Sprouts   82
    Pizza Dip   83
    Baked Beans with Nachos   85
    Roasted Parsnips   87
    Pancetta Brussels Sprouts   88

DESSERTS   89
    S'mores Delight   89
    Cinnamon Apple Cake   91

APPENDIX

Cooking Conversion Charts

1. Measuring Equivalent Chart

Type	Imperial	Imperial	Metric
Weight	1 dry ounce		28g
	1 pound	16 dry ounces	0.45 kg
Volume	1 teaspoon		5 ml
	1 dessert spoon	2 teaspoons	10 ml
	1 tablespoon	3 teaspoons	15 ml
	1 Australian tablespoon	4 teaspoons	20 ml
	1 fluid ounce	2 tablespoons	30 ml
	1 cup	16 tablespoons	240 ml
	1 cup	8 fluid ounces	240 ml
	1 pint	2 cups	470 ml
	1 quart	2 pints	0.95 l
	1 gallon	4 quarts	3.8 l
Length	1 inch		2.54 cm

* Numbers are rounded to the closest equivalent

2. Oven Temperature Equivalent Chart

Fahrenheit (°F)	Celsius (°C)	Gas Mark
220	100	
225	110	1/4
250	120	1/2
275	140	1
300	150	2
325	160	3
350	180	4
375	190	5
400	200	6
425	220	7
450	230	8
475	250	9
500	260	

* Celsius (°C) = T (°F)-32] * 5/9
** Fahrenheit (°F) = T (°C) * 9/5 + 32
*** Numbers are rounded to the closest equivalent

Printed in Great Britain
by Amazon